Gurdon Buck

A contribution to the surgical therapeutics of the air-passages, illustrated by two cases

Gurdon Buck

A contribution to the surgical therapeutics of the air-passages, illustrated by two cases

ISBN/EAN: 9783337809447

Printed in Europe, USA, Canada, Australia, Japan

Cover: Foto ©ninafisch / pixelio.de

More available books at **www.hansebooks.com**

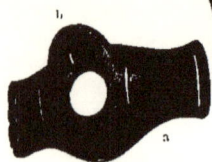

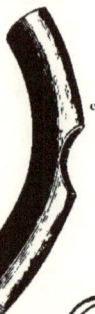

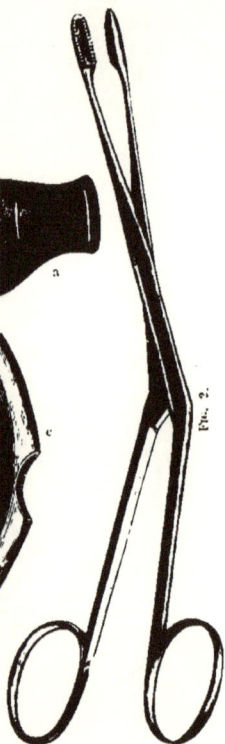

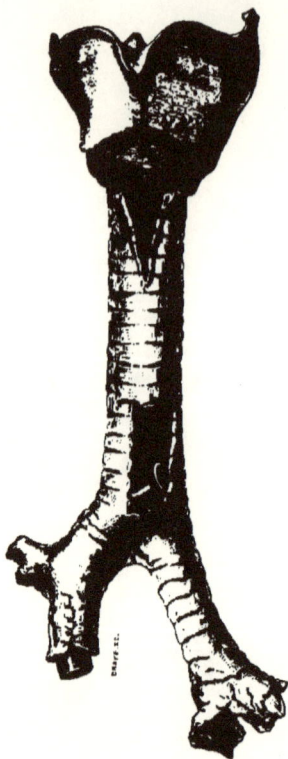

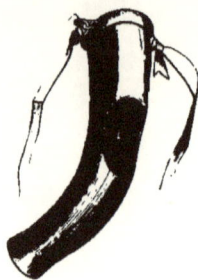

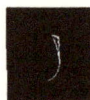

Fig. 1.

Fig. 2.

Fig. 3.

Fig. 4.

Fig. 5.

A CONTRIBUTION

TO THE

SURGICAL THERAPEUTICS OF THE AIR-PASSAGES.

ILLUSTRATED BY TWO CASES.

By GURDON BUCK, M.D.,

SURGEON TO NEW YORK HOSPITAL, ST. LUKE'S HOSPITAL, ETC., ETC.

CASE

Removal of a Morbid Growth from the Cavity of the Larynx by Laryngo-Tracheotomy, subsequent escape of a hard rubber trachea tube into the right bronchus, and its removal by operation.

JOHN MCGIVNEY, æt. 38, native of Ireland, coachman, admitted into St. Luke's Hospital, April 15, 1870, with laryngeal trouble, of which the following is a description :—His voice is reduced to a hoarse whisper; his respiration is labored and obstructed alike in inspiration and expiration, and is accompanied with laryngeal resonance. Dyspnœa is aggravated by going up stairs, incautious swallowing, and other disturbing causes. Inspection of the fauces detects no other appearance than a general paleness of the surface, and digital exploration ascertains that the epiglottis is normal in size and position. Patient is thin in flesh and of sallow complexion, and has continued at his occupation up to the time of his admission into the hospital. He persistently denies any venereal antecedents, and has had no inflammatory attack affecting the air-passages. For years past his ordinary colds, he says, have been accompanied by violent coughing. About three or four months ago his voice began to be affected, and his breathing to be disturbed. Both troubles have gradually increased up to the present time.

Externally the region of the larynx presents no change in its appearance, nor does outward pressure have any particular effect. Patient's sensations refer to the larynx as the seat of his trouble.

The absence of all local inflammatory symptoms, together with the presence of symptoms of laryngeal obstruction, which have developed themselves gradually, point to the existence of a growth in the interior of the larynx as the cause of the trouble. This conclusion was confirmed by laryngoscopic examinations made by different experts. A growth (not papilliform) was seen in the cavity of the larynx below the vocal cords. Up to the 23d of April palliative treatment was used, but without affording any relief; on the contrary, the dyspnœa increased, and suffocating exacerbations became more severe and threatening. The danger of suffocation seemed so urgent that it was decided to resort to tracheotomy without further delay. Accordingly, a consultation having been summoned, the operation was performed at seven o'clock the same evening, and without etherization.

An incision was made in the median line from the thyroid notch downward to the sternal notch, and the tissues divided successively until the crico-thyroid membrane, the cricoid cartilage, and the three upper tracheal rings were laid bare. The struggling efforts of the patient during these proceedings aggravated very much the dyspnœa, so that in the extreme movements of respiration the cricoid cartilage would descend nearly to the level of the upper margin of the sternum. The crico-thyroid membrane itself, under pressure of the end of the finger, seemed very unyielding, as if there were resistance from within the laryngeal cavity. The operation having been unavoidably protracted, the dyspnœa had become very urgent, and suffocation seemed impending, when, without further delay, the trachea was opened by plunging a scalpel, with its back downward, in between the second and third tracheal ring, and cutting first upward through the cricoid cartilage, and then transversely along its upper margin, thus giving the opening a letter **T** shape.

Instantly the air rushed into the trachea with a whizzing sound, and on the insertion of a trachea tube the respiration soon became tranquil. The patient, who had long been deprived of rest, fell asleep before being removed to his ward. Nothing was attempted for the removal of the intra-laryngeal growth until the following day, April 24th, at 2 o'clock P.M., when a second operation was performed, with the aid of the other surgeons of the hospital and several invited professional friends.

Patient had passed a comfortable night, and was in good spirits and ready to be again operated on. It was now proposed to lay open the larynx in front, and expose its cavity for the purpose of removing the morbid growth from within. After etherization an incision was continued up to the os hyoides, and the thyroid cartilage exposed. A grooved director was passed into the cavity of the larynx, through the existing opening from below upward, and served to conduct the distal blade of a pair of scissors, curved edgewise, with which the thyroid cartilage was divided vertically through its notch, special care being taken to make the section exactly in the median line, and thereby avoid the vocal cords. The incision was also continued upward through the thyro-hyoid membrane. This permitted the two halves of the larynx to be drawn wide apart, exposing its cavity to full view. At first the entire cavity seemed to be filled up with the growth;—but a further careful examination ascertained that it occupied the right wall of the larynx, and involved the ventricle and both vocal cords underneath which it had originated, and which, together with the neighboring lining membrane, it had elevated and pushed inward so as considerably to encroach upon and narrow the laryngeal cavity. A small prolongation of the growth, somewhat pedunculated, emerged from the ventricle, between the cords, and protruded further into the cavity of the larynx. To remove the mass entire, an incision was made circumscribing its base and extending half an inch below the inferior vocal cord. It was carried down to the cartilage, from the surface of which the whole mass was detached from below upward. After dividing its connection above, it was found that the right arytenoid cartilage had been excised, and formed a part of the mass removed. No troublesome hemorrhage followed. Two or three points of suspicious appearance on the surface of the wound were touched with the actual cautery. Two thread sutures were inserted into the tissues covering the thyroid cartilage, to hold its cut edges in accurate coaptation, and the edges of the wound were brought together by two pin sutures above and one below the tube. In addition to these there were several thread sutures. A trachea tube of extra length was found necessary, owing to the depth of the trachea. Patient's subsequent progress was so favorable that in three or four days after the operation he left his bed and continued up and about. After the subsidence of the swelling he wore a hard rubber tube of medium size, corked at its outer end. His respiration was perfectly easy, and his voice remained very much the same as before the first operation. A copious viscid secretion was ejected through the tube by coughing.

May 10*th*.—The wound is entirely healed above and below the tube. The tumor removed was subjected to a microscopic examination, and found to be made up of small, round, nucleated cells, about the size of lymph cells, imbedded in a tolerably abundant fibrous stroma. The growth was of a pretty firm consistence.

Patient continued to do well up to Wednesday night, May 25th, when a very extraordinary accident occurred. Having gone to bed as well as usual, he was waked out of sleep about ten o'clock by violent coughing and struggling for breath. Soon, however, he became quiet and fell asleep, but was again waked up later in the night by a second attack similar to, but less violent than, the first. He now discovered that his trachea tube had disappeared, and, alarmed at the discovery, sent for the house-surgeon, who on examination found, to his great surprise, that the tube had disappeared, while the collar-piece (Fig. 1, a) which had supported the outer end of the tube, and to which the tape fastenings were attached, was undisturbed. The cork which had closed the outer orifice of the tube also remained *in situ*, occupying as it did a rim (Fig. 1, b) which formed a piece separate from the tube itself, but joined to it by a shallow-threaded screw. A separation had taken place at this joint, and the tube (Fig. 1, c) had dropped off, while the rim was still held in place by the collar-piece. The house-surgeon passed a probe several inches down the trachea, and a probang down the œsophagus, but encountered nothing. Patient believing that the tube was lodged in the larynx, from a feeling of soreness in that part, the house-surgeon passed a finger of one hand into the larynx from above, through the mouth, and a finger of the other hand through the opening in the trachea below, and made them meet in the cavity of the larynx. He also had the patient elevated, with the feet upward and the head downward, thumping him at the same time between the scapulæ. At the regular visit on the following day, May 26th, patient continued perfectly free from any disturbing symptoms, and had no consciousness of any effect from the accident. Such a perfect state of quietude was thought to be incompatible with the presence of the tube in the air-passages, and it seemed a more probable conclusion that in the first paroxysm of coughing provoked by the presence of the intruding body, the tube had been projected into the fauces, and that the patient in his half-awake, half-asleep condition had swallowed it. Directions were accordingly given to watch his stools, in the hope of finding the tube.

The same uniform quiet condition persisted up to Wednesday, June 1st, when Dr. J. R. Leaming, one of the attending physicians, had his attention called to the case, and instituted a careful auscultatory examination of the patient's chest.

The doctor has kindly furnished me the following memorandum of his examination :—" In the left lung were signs denoting chronic pulmonary disease and the presence of viscid mucus, but no foreign body.

" In the right lung the breath sounds were peculiar in pitch and sonoriety, the respiratory murmur was everywhere distinct, though feeble, notwithstanding the peculiarity of the breath sound. This peculiarity had one point of greatest intensity, confined to the upper part of the interscapular space, about one inch and a half long vertically, and one inch wide, on the right side of the spine. Here the breath sound was heard as a modification of bronchial breathing, of equal length in inspiration and expiration, and of the same pitch in both. It was A in the musical scale.

" This was evidence of the immediate presence of the missing

tube, with the air passing through it. The lung immediately
underneath the upper part of the interscapular space is supplied
with air by the upper branch of the first division of the right
bronchus, and the tube must have been engaged in this bronchus to have caused the maximum intensity of sound at this
place. The length of the first division of the bronchus is not
quite half an inch, consequently the upper end of the tube
must have extended through the right bronchus into the
trachea."

Having confidence in the accuracy of Dr. Leaming's examination, I directed notices to be issued for a consultation on the
following day, Thursday, June 2d, at three o'clock. Dr. L.
had already repeated his examination, and corroborated his conclusions of the day before. The patient, moreover, admitted
that his breathing was not as satisfactory now as it had been,
and auscultation showed that the respiratory sound had become
less distinct over the right lung than over the left. My col-
leagues of the hospital and several other medical friends present examined the patient carefully, and corroborated the condition already ascertained. They also expressed their approbation
of my proposal to attempt the removal of the tube by a surgical
operation. It was performed as follows :—

Patient having been etherized, and the trachea tube removed,
an incision was made from the lower margin of the existing
opening, along the median line, to a point two inches below
the sternal notch. The tissues subjacent to the skin were
successively divided until the trachea was laid bare to the
extent of one inch. To facilitate as much as possible the
stretching apart of the edges of the wound, the incision of the
skin and soft parts subjacent was continued a short distance
upward above the opening. The exposed trachea was now
divided from below upward, so as to communicate with, and
very considerably enlarge, the existing opening. A needle
threaded with a coarse ligature was passed through the edges
of the wound, at opposite points, so as to include the cut edges
of the trachea, and the ends of the ligatures tied to form
loops with which to stretch wide apart the tracheal opening.
While this was done by assistants, a flexible silver probe, seven
inches long, fixed in a handle, and slightly curved in its whole

length, and bent into a small hook at its point, was passed down into the trachea, with its point directed to the right side. After passing to the depth of seven inches, the tube was encountered and its contact distinctly felt and appreciated by several of those present. Probably the end of the probe had passed through and beyond the tube, inasmuch as my colleague, Prof. H. B. Sands, having introduced his finger immediately afterward, announced that he could just reach it with the end of his forefinger. With the end of my little finger I now ascertained that the end of the tube presented itself obliquely to the axis of the trachea. I thereupon introduced a long and slender dressing forceps, bent edgewise at an obtuse angle (see Fig. 2), and with it seized and brought away the tube. The wound was closed as after the previous operation, and a trachea tube replaced. A copious expectoration of viscid mucus followed the operation, but without any bloody discoloration. The subsequent progress was favorable, and at the end of three or four days patient was again up and about the ward.

June 17*th.*—The wound has healed perfectly above and below the tube, and all inflammatory swelling of the surface has disappeared. Patient is quite free from cough and disturbance of respiration; his voice continues very much the same as before the first operation.

Desirous of returning to his home, patient was discharged wearing the tube.

On Monday, June 27th, he was subjected to a laryngoscopic examination by my friend Dr. F. Simrock, who has kindly furnished me the following report :—" Quite contrary to my expectation, I found the glottis quite patulous while the breathing is going on. The mobility of the left vocal cord is normal, and its excursion in approaching the right side of the larynx exceeds the median line. There is some ulceration yet to be seen at the former place of the right vocal cord, and it is impossible to see how far down toward the trachea the ulcerative process reaches. I would not have the least hesitation in leaving out the tube."

On Friday, July 1st, the trachea tube was left out entirely. Exuberant granulations, which had sprung up around the orifice of the opening through which the tube passed, were pared away close to the skin, and the fresh-cut surface freely touched with nitrate of silver. A compress, spread with cerate, was applied over the opening, and secured in place by narrow strips of adhesive plaster.

July 7th.—Patient was exhibited at a meeting of the Academy of Medicine; the opening is reduced to a very small-sized chink.

26th.—The opening is entirely closed, a linear cicatrix in the median line of the neck marks the seat of the operation. Patient is directed to extend his neck to its utmost capacity several times daily for the purpose of lengthening the cicatrix.

Oct. 14th, '70.—Patient was examined by several medical gentlemen at St. Luke's Hospital. His general health is excellent. His voice has improved. Some words are now articulated in a clear tone, whereas previously his articulation was exclusively in a rough and hoarse whisper. Dec. 7th, '70.— Patient's voice has further improved. His articulation has become loud, though still hoarse, and is no longer whispering. Vowels and consonants are articulated with equal facility. He is unable to raise his voice above its ordinary pitch. His respiration is easy and natural, and he is free from cough or expectoration.

The tube extracted in this case measures separately two inches and five-eighths in length on its convex side, and two inches on its concave; its distal end is three-eighths of an inch in diameter, and its proximal end, where it joins the collar-plate, one-half inch outside measurement. Its convex side is perforated at its middle by a fenestrum one-half an inch in its longitudinal diameter. (See Fig. 1, c.)

By resorting to the cadaver it was found that the tube placed in the right bronchus could not be made to lodge entirely within the bronchus; its proximal end remained in the trachea at its bifurcation, and when placed with its convexity toward the right side the proximal end of the tube presented itself obliquely upward, which was the position it occupied at the time of the operation, as recognized by Prof. Sands as well as myself. When, however, the position of the tube was changed so that its convexity looked to the opposite side, toward the median line, the proximal end then looked directly upward toward the larynx, and its convex side near the extremity was no longer within reach of the finger, as it was in the first position. This is shown in Fig. 3.

The state of complete quietude following the first disturbing effects of this extraordinary accident, and persisting as it did for one week afterward, may be explained by the fact that the tubular form of the foreign body, largely perforated in its middle, caused very little or no obstruction to the passage of air. Its form, too, being curved, both ends of the tube rested against the walls of the passage in which it was lodged, and tended to hold it at rest. This condition of quietude, however, had reached its limit. The patient on the day of the operation, just one week after the accident, began to experience some difficulty in respiration, and the respiratory murmur had become more indistinct over the right lung. A longer delay of the operation would no doubt have developed increasing manifestations of obstruction.

THE OPERATION.

The introduction of forceps and other instruments into the trachea and bronchi, through an opening in the neck, for the removal of foreign bodies has been successfully practised in numerous instances recorded by different authors. The introduction of the finger, however, into the trachea, for the purpose of ascertaining the situation of a foreign body, is a proceeding altogether new within the knowledge of the author. The facility of this operation in the present case, and the practical advantage of it in guiding to the prompt and easy removal of the foreign body, furnished a very suggestive practical lesson to all present on the occasion.

My worthy colleague, Prof. H. B. Sands, to whom belongs the priority in digital exploration of the interior of the trachea, joins me in not only sanctioning but recommending the practice as safe, and as affording a sure guide to further proceedings for the removal of the body we are in search of. Its application is so momentary as scarcely to occasion any impediment to respiration. It may be directed not only downward toward the bifurcation, as in the present case, but also upwards through the larynx, to ascertain the condition of the vocal cords and ventricles, and also of the epiglottis and its surroundings. It would be of special advantage where a foreign body, as has often happened, has become lodged in one of the ventricles.

The operation performed in this case proved to be well adapted to the employment of digital exploration. The opening in the trachea must necessarily be very free, and a vertical incision should be made of at least one inch in length, commencing at the lower edge of the cricoid cartilage, and dividing the five upper rings of the trachea. To make this opening capable of the greatest degree of dilatation, a transverse incision should also be carried across its upper extremity, between the first tracheal ring and the cricoid cartilage, to the extent of half an inch on either side. (See Fig. 3.) A ligature passed through the opposite edges of the wound, and including the tissues immediately in contact with the trachea, but without perforating it, with the ends tied together so as to form a loop, affords the most convenient means of stretching the edges of the opening apart. The division of the isthmus of the thyroid body, necessarily involved in this operation, need not be dreaded. The author, in his numerous operations for tracheotomy, has never had any special difficulty from hemorrhage from this part, nor has he ever taken the precaution to previously ligate the isthmus on either side of the median line and then cut between the ligatures. Such a precaution might easily be taken, and would be a complete security against hemorrhage.

After previous digital exploration, the forceps best adapted to seize a foreign body in the trachea below, or in the larynx above, is the one represented by Fig. 2.

Should the foreign body be lodged in either bronchus, it might still be reached, and though not seized, it might be dislodged and expelled by coughing.

REMARKS.—We have in the case just narrated a rare and exceptional instance of a foreign body getting into the air-passages without passing through the larynx. The few examples on record of this mode of entrance have been most frequently those occurring in gunshot wounds. A memorable exception is, however, reported by De la Martinière, in vol. v. of Mém. de l'Acad. Royale de Chirurgie, p. 346, of a copper pin fifteen lines in length that pierced the trachea just below the cricoid cartilage, transfixing the tube and penetrating its opposite wall. Having no head, the pin buried itself below the surface of the skin at its entrance.

In Professor G. D. Gross's very thorough and able Treatise on Foreign Bodies in the Air-Passages, he enumerates a great variety of substances which have got into the air-passages. Among those of a vegetable nature were beans, grains of corn, seeds of different kinds, pits of fruits, nut-shells, ears of grass and rye, cockleburs, etc. Among those of an animal nature were bits of meat, bone, shell, claws, quill, teeth, human and animal, besides a variety of other substances. Buttons, pins, needles, beads, shot, coin, nails, and other metallic substances were also on the list.

M. Bonrdillat, in an article, "Observations pour servir à l'Histoire des Corps Étrangers dans les Voies Aériennes," in *Gazette Médicale de Paris*, No. 7, 15 Fevrier, 1868, has collected three hundred cases of foreign bodies in the air-passages, of which seventy-eight were cases of beans, sixteen of cherry pits, nineteen of prune pits, eighteen of pieces of bone, five of coin, nine of teeth, six of water-melon seeds, besides a great variety of other substances. Neither author furnishes any instance of a trachea tube dropping into the air-passages, as in the case now reported. In his researches, however, the author has discovered one other case, recorded in the *Brit. Med. Journal*, Feb. 15, 1868, p. 141, by J. Waters, M.B., Reigate, England, which is given below entire.

T. W., aged 40, tailor, twelve years ago had tracheotomy performed for disease of the larynx and glottis following fever. He had worn the tube ever since, not being able to do without it. The voice had been distinct, but husky. On March 22, 1867, at 8.30 A.M., while he was attempting to remove the tube, as he was accustomed to do for cleansing, the rim came off and he could not get hold of the cylinder. When I saw him shortly afterwards I could see the tube at the bottom of the wound. I went down stairs to get instruments from the carriage, and to ask Dr. Holman to assist me. When I returned the tube had slipped down the trachea, and could only be felt by a bent probe at a distance of five inches from the external opening, to the right. Respiration was imperfect over the right side of the chest, perfect on the left. Attacks of dyspnœa were at times moderately severe, and cough very troublesome. Inversion was tried, with smart blows on the front and back, without altering the position of the tube. At 3 P.M., having obtained a pair of long-curved forceps, we resolved to make further attempts to remove the tube. A stilette, bent at the end, was first introduced, and caught something which seemed like the tube, but on making traction, smart bright hemorrhage came rather freely from the tracheal wound, so the hook was disengaged and withdrawn. Chloroform was then administered over the mouth and trachea. It excited him much at first, but he soon went under its influence; the long forceps were then introduced and the tube was felt, but it could not be caught; bloody mucus came freely from the mouth and wound, and he retched freely. The respiration became so much impaired that the chloroform had to be given up, and time given him to eject the accumulation in his air-passages. This condition being somewhat perilous, when he had sufficiently recovered I made a fresh examination, and found the tube rather more than five inches down, and to the left. After one or two failures, the tube was seized with the long forceps and drawn to the wound, where it stuck, and while Dr. Holman was enlarging the opening to admit its removal it slipped back. I managed, however, to catch it again immediately, fortunately, this time, in the long axis, and it was readily removed, and found to be filled with mucous membrane. After the removal he complained merely of being weary and of some soreness of the chest. He suffered, during the attempts at removal, merely distress from obstruction to the breathing. His recovery was very rapid, and in a few days he was able to resume his work.

An important point worthy of notice in this case is the condition of the voice after the removal of the vocal cord and arytenoid eminence of the right side. In this respect the case is believed to be quite unique, and without example in the records of surgery.

The following report of the condition of the interior of the larynx, as ascertained by a laryngoscopic examination made by R. F. Weir, M.D., has been furnished by him :—

"The left vocal cord is drawn beyond the median line toward the opposite side in phonation. The cicatrix presents a sharp, curved line, running backward, and appearing to be attached to the opposite arytenoid cartilage, and lost in the adjacent pharyngeal tissues. This bridle-like cicatrix moves slightly to meet the remaining vocal cord in phonation. Below is a reddish projection, and still farther below, and anterior, is a yellowish mass that I take to be the cicatrix of the trachea.

"R. F. Weir.

"Dec. 13, 1870."

Case II.

A fish-bone lodged in the larynx during a period of fourteen years.—A trachea tube inserted after laryngo-tracheotomy, and worn twelve years and then dispensed with.

On the 22d May, 1855, Mrs. F. C. J., æt. 25, daughter of a physician residing at N. R., while eating small fish at dinner had a bone lodged in her throat, which at once caused great disturbance and violent efforts of coughing and hawking to dislodge the foreign body. Her father improvised a probang and passed it down the œsophagus, and resorted to various other measures for her relief, but without success. She could reach the bone on the left side of the throat with her left forefinger, and perceived that the end of the bone pointed upward. The same evening, at about 9 o'clock, while taking some food, the bone became dislodged, and complete relief followed, to her great joy and that of her family. For eight days she continued well, with the exception of slight remaining soreness, and then began to cough. As she had been somewhat exposed in a visit to the city, the cough was attributed to her having taken cold. Soon the cough became croupy and sonorous, and very frequent, especially at night. Her husband was struck with the croupy character of the cough from the outset. Soon the voice began to be affected with hoarseness, at first only at night when suffering from attacks of dyspnœa; subsequently, however, the hoarseness became constant. Suffocative attacks at night increased in severity, and sometimes were very alarming. The use of opiates at bedtime, such as Dover's Powder, or M'Munn's Elixir of Opium, became indispensable, and would often keep her easy for the night. She writes of her own case as follows:—" On the night of 7th July, 1855, I was seized with severe coughing, accompanied by a great sense of oppression, together with much distress and aching about the throat. Warm fomentations and inhalations were tried, but without any decided relief. The distress continued for seven hours, gradually diminishing as daylight appeared. Since that time I have been constantly subject to similar attacks, varying greatly in frequency and degree. Sometimes they would return

as often as once a week, usually taking about two days to reach
their height and pass away. At other times several weeks
have elapsed without more than a slight return of the difficulty.
During the most severe paroxysms the sufferings were intense,
the breathing was hard and labored, accompanied by a sense of
suffocation, which was greatly aggravated by the least excite-
ment, or even by any motion of the body such as walking
across the room, &c. The effort of going up stairs would be
followed by very great oppression, so as to be at times almost
beyond endurance. The distress generally increased at the
approach of night; the darkness seemed to aggravate the difficulty. It was also necessary often to maintain an erect posture
in bed, with the head inclined forwards, being the only way to
obtain relief in breathing. The last attack of the kind was on
the 8th January, 1858. After a day of severe and almost inces-
sant coughing, the difficulty of breathing became very manifest
as night drew near, and when aggravated by coughing it almost
amounted to suffocation. I could not endure the darkness, and
was obliged to keep the gas burning through the night. The
cough was kept partially under control by means of an anodyne,
without which it seemed to me I could not live till morning.
The distress diminished as daylight appeared, and the next
day found me more comfortable." There was nothing visible or
tangible in the throat. Deglutition was easy. Sometimes she
felt pain darting through the throat, and also soreness in a particular spot on the left side when pressure was made with the
finger over the thyroid cartilage. She has had no fever at any
time, has felt in other respects well, and had never previously been
subject to cough or throat trouble. The cough has been without
expectoration from the first. July 7th, 1855, nearly seven
weeks after the accident, I saw Mrs. J. for the first time, in
consultation with her father, her uncle, and Dr. Voris, her attending physician. The conclusion arrived at, as the result of
our consultation, was, that Mrs. J.'s ailment was unconnected
with the accident of the fish-bone. An application of leeches
over the larynx, a mild mercurial course, alum emetics, and inhalations of vapor were advised and tried, but were followed by
only temporary benefit. The mercurial was afterwards resumed,
and blisters applied over the larynx. Anodynes were also given

at bedtime. No permanent benefit followed; on the contrary, her condition grew steadily worse. Dyspnœa became constant by day as well as by night, and was aggravated by every exertion. Mrs. J. having come to the city, a second consultation was held on the 29th September, 1855, in which Drs. Cammann, Willard Parker, and John Watson joined the original consultants. Each gentleman visited and examined the patient separately the day before. After a full discussion it was unanimously agreed that the origin and persistence of the symptoms depended on the presence of the fish-bone in or near the larynx, and that a surgical operation was the only resource from which relief was to be expected.

From this time onward Mrs. J. continued to suffer from cough and suffocative attacks with varying degrees of severity. At no time was she free from hoarseness, though in her best moments it was slight. Breathing, even when most tranquil, was accompanied with an audible laryngeal resonance. She continued to be without expectoration, except on the supervention of an ordinary cold, when the sputa presented the ordinary appearance of mucus.

Her suffocative attacks recurred frequently at night, and often with an alarming severity. Her general health suffered no material change till the end of the summer of 1857, when, on the 22d August, I was again requested to visit her at her father's residence in the country, in company with her uncle, Prof. J. M. S. The night previous she had had an attack of unusual severity, which had so much alarmed her father that he had sent to the city for assistance. We found her relieved of her urgent symptoms, but still suffering from the exhausting effects of the last night's attack. From this time till early in the following month of January (1858), when she came to the city to reside, Mrs. J. felt that her general health was steadily deteriorating; her suffocative attacks had become more frequent and severe, and during the intervals her relief was only partial. It should be remarked that during the whole progress of her ailment Mrs. J. has experienced a circumscribed soreness, referred to the left side of the larynx, over the thyroid cartilage. The failure of her general health, and the aggravation of her symptoms experienced during the past three or four months, have brought Mrs. J. to feel not only willing to submit to an operation, but desirous of it. Her husband shares the same feeling, and her parents also are convinced that it is the only resource from which relief can be expected.

On the 7th January, 1858, another consultation was held, in which Dr. Cammann, Professors A. Clark and Joseph M. Smith, as physicians, and Professor W. Parker and Dr. J. Watson, as surgeons, took part with the writer. Each consultant visited and examined the patient separately before the consultation.

After a free expression of opinion and discussion, the following conclusions were arrived at :—

1. That there was no evidence of tuberculosis or other disease in the lungs or elsewhere.

2. That Mrs. J.'s condition is to be attributed to the continued presence of the fish-bone swallowed in the month of May, 1855, all her symptoms dating their origin from that occurrence; and inasmuch as a sore spot has uniformly been felt, and referred to the left side of the thyroid cartilage, and to a point corresponding to the situation of the left ventricle of the larynx, it is thought possible that the bone is imbedded in the ventricle.

3. That inasmuch as no relief had been afforded by any medical treatment hitherto employed, but, on the contrary, the patient is steadily growing worse, and is in constant danger of suffocation from the increasing laryngismus, a surgical operation is required, and should be resorted to without delay.

4. That in order to expose the interior of the larynx, and to remove the foreign body supposed to be lodged in it, and also to provide, if necessary, for the establishment of a tube permanently in the trachea, with the view of thereby leaving the larynx itself at rest, the operation of laryngo-tracheotomy is to be preferred in this case. On the 10th January, at 10 o'clock, another consultation was held, when the same consultants were present, with Professor A. H. Stevens added to their number. The former conclusion was confirmed, and two o'clock of the same day was appointed for the performance of the operation.

OPERATION.

Patient was placed on a narrow bed facing a window, and the bedstead elevated at its head so as to form an inclined plane. Ether having been administered, an incision was made in the median line, from the os hyoides to the third tracheal ring, and the tissues successively divided till the cartilages were laid bare. The hemorrhage, which was moderate, was allowed to cease before incising the larynx. The crico-thyroid membrane was first pierced in the median line, and the incision continued upward from the upper edge of the cricoid cartilage through the lower half of the thyroid cartilage. At this moment the air rushing in through the opening, the lungs seemed as though taken by surprise, and for an instant intermitted their action. In order to afford prompt and free access of air to the lungs, I immediately extended the incision downward through the cricoid cartilage and the two upper tracheal rings, and stretched the edges of the opening apart. As soon as the respiration had become quietly established through the wound, I divided the upper half of the thyroid cartilage very exactly in the median line through the notch. The next step was to make a thorough inspection of the interior of the larynx, especially of the left ventricle. The attempts to do this, by stretching apart the edges of the wound, excited a good deal of disturbance, such as coughing, suffocation, etc., so that we were compelled frequently to desist and allow patient to recover herself. After an hour and a half occupied in these proceedings, patient became so much exhausted that it was thought most prudent to postpone further examination to the following day. Respiration being performed with entire facility through the wound, a tube was not inserted. The examination, so far as we had been able to make it, ascertained the existence of a spot, of the size of a small split pea, on the inner surface of the cricoid cartilage, posteriorly and to the left side, where the mucous membrane was wanting and the surface was of a deep red or purplish color. The cartilage was not exposed, nor could a probe detect any track leading from it. The ventricles appeared to be in a normal condition, and the finger passed upward through the glottis could perceive nothing abnormal. The wound was left open, and kept covered with compresses wet in tepid water. The pulse, which had risen to 120, subsided to 100. The succeeding twenty-four hours were passed comfortably. A viscid mucous expectoration, stained with blood, was expelled through the wound by coughing. On the following day, at 12 o'clock, the examination was resumed in the presence of the same gentlemen as attended the day before. The parts had now become very sore from inflammation, which rendered the examination very painful, especially as ether could not be administered. The divided edges of the larynx were stretched apart, and the interior surface carefully inspected. The spot already noticed was seen, and its appearance verified as described above. No pus was observed on its surface or in its neighborhood. A thin layer of lymph exudation, the product of recent inflammation, coated the posterior surface of the laryngeal cavity. In order to establish a tube in the trachea, it was necessary to expose and divide two additional trachea rings at the lower angle of the wound. After doing this the upper ring was detached from the lower edge of the cricoid cartilage to the extent of two lines on either side of the vertical slit, and a triangular piece clipped away with scissors from each angle, including portions of the three upper rings. This converted the vertical slit in the trachea into a triangular opening, with its base upward. A silver trachea tube was then inserted, and secured by tapes passed around the neck. The wound above the tube was closed in the following manner:—

1st. By a single suture, inserted into the muscular and aponeurotic tissues covering the thyroid cartilage on either side of the median incision. This held the opposite edges of the cartilage in exact coaptation. It was observed before introducing this suture that in every act of deglutition the cut edges of the thyroid cartilage were drawn apart by the action of the constrictor muscles of the pharynx.

2d. Four interrupted thread sutures were inserted into the edges of the integument, between the tube and upper angle of the wound.

3d. The whole was supported by strips of adhesive plaster crossing from one side of the neck to the other, between the sutures. Before closing the larynx, the ulcerated spot noticed on its inner surface was freely touched with nitrate of silver.

The constitutional disturbance following the operation was at no time very considerable. Within one week the pulse subsided to below 80. The cough was variable, sometimes severe and in paroxysms, and at other times suspended for long intervals. The expectoration ceased to be bloody after the first twenty-four hours, and during the first five or six days was opaque, viscid, and rather copious, and then gradually became transparent, frothy, and much less in quantity. During the first week the tube required to be changed twice in twenty-four hours; after that, but once a day. There was no appearance of pus at any time in the expectoration, nor was there any feeling of soreness around the track of the tube. The respiration through the tube was from the first perfectly free. The wound healed above the tube by first intention, and at the end of three and a half weeks it had also healed around the lower side. Three weeks after the operation a tube, perforated at its middle on the convex side, was worn, and with it the patient enjoyed the use of her voice by corking the outer orifice of the tube. At first articulation was performed in a hoarse whisper, and respiration through the larynx was attended with some effort; but gradually the obstacles diminished, and at date of Feb. 13, 1858, Mrs. J. wears the tube for hours, and is not sensible of any difference in breathing with or without the cork inserted. Her general health is greatly improved.

Under date of July 13, 1869, Mrs. J., at my request, furnished me the following statement :—" In regard to the condition of my health while wearing the tube, I can say there has been a manifest improvement. The principal difficulty has been an inability to take any violent exercise or motion. The effort of going up-stairs, or making any ascent, is followed by more or less difficulty of breathing. The cough has never left me, though, unless aggravated by cold, it does not cause much inconvenience. There have been occasional returns of the suffocative attacks, though at intervals of several months, similar to the former ones, but varying in degree. Wearing the tube has caused very little discomfort; on the contrary, I am hardly conscious of its presence. There has been no constant soreness in the region of the tube, though occasionally the outer surface around the opening through which it passes into the windpipe has become swollen and inflamed, causing a good deal of inconvenience. I have always kept two tubes, one for the day, the other for the night, and have changed and cleaned them regularly morning and evening." During the long period of twelve years that Mrs. J. was obliged to wear the trachea tube she abated nothing of her accustomed activity in the discharge of her ordinary duties. In the summer season she often accompanied her friends on distant travelling excursions. The tube being concealed from view by the arrangement of her neck-dress, there was nothing to betray her condition to casual observers. A slight huskiness of voice, and that by no means conspicuous, was all that was noticeable.

One morning in the month of June, 1869, Mrs. J. having, as usual, removed the tube to cleanse it, noticed something sticking to its outer surface, on the left side, near the fenestrum, to which she called her father's attention, and which, on minute examination, proved to be a small fish-bone, about five-eighths of an inch in length, curved, flattened, and triangular at one end, but growing smaller and tapering at the other end.

For several weeks previous to this occurrence she had suffered from a frequent accumulation around the inner end of the tube and the opposite surface of the trachea, of viscid, tenacious secretion, that would obstruct breathing and provoke violent coughing paroxysms for its expulsion. Often she was obliged to remove these accumulations by seizing the matter with a forceps inserted into the opening, after first removing the tube. Sometimes they came away in a tubular shape, and were of very tough consistency. Complete relief always followed their removal.

The important question of dispensing with the trachea tube now urged itself upon our consideration. Mrs. J. and her family naturally felt great hesitation in making the experiment, fearing as they did that the closure of the opening might narrow the calibre of the trachea to such a degree as to obstruct respiration. This fear was met by the consideration that the tube itself occupied more space in the trachea than would be lost by the contraction consequent upon the closure of the opening, if any took place. The author could also cite from his own observation a case in which tracheotomy having been performed, and a triangular portion of the two upper tracheal rings having been excised, the tube, after being worn for several months, had worked its way gradually up into the larynx. At a post-mortem examination, no trace of loss of substance could be detected ; the rings of the trachea were identified and found complete from the cricoid cartilage downward. The specimen is preserved in the Pathological Cabinet of the New York Hospital. The reproduction of the tracheal rings seemed thus to be conclusively established. The question of removal of the tube, however, continued in abeyance till January 21, 1870, when Mrs. J., having come to the city for the winter, was disposed to undertake the experiment. Before doing so, however, it was thought best to ascertain the condition of the interior of the larynx by a thorough examination with the laryngoscope. This was done very satisfactorily by my friend Dr. F. Simrock, not only by the application of the mirror above through the fauces, but also below through the opening in the neck. It was ascertained that there was no thickening of the vocal cords or other parts, nor any contraction of the laryngeal cavity. The inner surface of the trachea, seen through the opening in the neck, under exposure to sunlight, presented patches of adherent viscid exudation, such as, for some time previously, had accumulated and occasioned obstruction of the respiration. To expel these accumulated secretions violent paroxysms of coughing were provoked, as already noticed. Encouraged still further by the result of the laryngoscopic examination, Mrs. J. now consented to the removal of the tube, which was left out. The opening situated in the median line of the neck, immediately below the cricoid cartilage, is about two-thirds of an inch in its vertical diameter, and five-eighths of an inch in its tranverse. Its margin is even and flush with the neighboring surface, which is somewhat sunken below the level of the surrounding parts. The skin is supple and movable up to the border of the opening. To facilitate the dislodgment and expulsion of the viscid tracheal secretion, patient was directed to inhale frequently the fumes from an infusion of catnip, and her father was to make an application to the trachea, through the opening, of a solution of nitrate of silver, of the strength of ten grains to the ounce, morning and evening. A compress, secured in place by strips of adhesive plaster, was worn over the opening to prevent the passage of air in respiration and coughing. Patient continued to be disturbed by the accumulation of viscid secretion in the trachea, and the cough provoked by it, till 21st February, when the external opening, after gradually diminishing in size, had become reduced to less than one-fourth its original dimensions, and the tracheal secretion had begun to make its way out through the larynx and mouth instead of through the tracheal opening.

May 28th.—Thirteen weeks having elapsed since the opening ceased to diminish in size, it was decided to perform an operation for its permanent closure.

OPERATION.

Ether having been administered, the margin of the orifice was pared away, and an incision extended a short distance above and below the opening. The edges of the skin were then dissected up on either side so as to permit broad raw surfaces to be confronted and secured in contact by means of three pin sutures, wound with cotton yarn, and intermediate thread sutures. Patient was directed, whenever she coughed, to make pressure with her fingers over the wound, so as to prevent the skin from being pushed away from the subjacent parts by the air seeking to force itself out through the tracheal opening.

June 2d.—Primary union has taken place except at two points, which permit an escape of air and frothy pus in small quantity. To close these, fresh sutures were inserted.

June 18th.—The closure of the wound is now complete, and the skin adherent to the subjacent parts. The opening in the trachea is not only closed by the skin covering it, but a gradual growth of the tracheal rings across the opening has been going on since the tube was left out. This process has been appreciable to the touch. A vertical slit, less than one-fourth of the size of the original opening, is all that now remains. Patient will now leave for the country, and will in a few days leave off the use of an elastic rubber band and compress which she has worn to support the parts.

June 30th.—Mrs. J. called to permit a final inspection. Everything about the wound is doing well. A vertical linear depression on the surface of the trachea is all that can be felt through the superjacent skin to mark the situation of the tracheal opening. The reproduction of the excised portion of tracheal rings appears to be complete. The parts involved in the operation are sunken in a hollow below the level of the surrounding surface. The tracheal secretion has lost its tough viscid character, and is much diminished in quantity. Respiration has suffered no impediment since the closure of the trachea.

Dec., 1870.—Mrs. J. continues to do well.

The question of chief interest suggested by this case relates to the whereabouts of the fish-bone during these long fourteen years of its sojourn in the larynx. The most satisfactory conclusion at which the author has been able to arrive in the retrospect of the history of the case is, that the bone, after producing immediate violent disturbance, was suddenly dislodged while Mrs. J. was taking food, and located itself in a situation where, for a few days, it ceased to provoke any disturbance. At length, however, it made its way into the left ventricle, where it lay concealed, and escaped detection when the cavity of the larnyx was laid open and explored. This conclusion is, perhaps, strengthened by the fact that a local soreness was felt by the patient during the whole course of her suffering on the left side of the larynx, and was referred by her to a spot corresponding to the situation of the left ventricle, at which spot outside digital pressure also produced pain. It will also be remembered that the fish-bone, when first discovered, was adhering to the surface of the trachea tube on its left side and near its middle. It is difficult to conceive of a substance like the fish-bone imbedding itself in the soft parts lining the cartilaginous parietes of the laryngeal cavity without ulceration and suppuration. The membrane lining the pouch-shaped ventricles, however, being lax and more or less wrinkled, the fish-bone, so minute as it was, might easily be concealed in its folds and escape detection. That it should have remained for so long a time is certainly very remarkable.

Fig. 4 shows the trachea tube worn by patient.

Fig. 5 the size and shape of the fish-bone discharged.